The Food Lord

Family Plants a Garden

Antonio Ford

The Food Lord

Family Plants a Garden

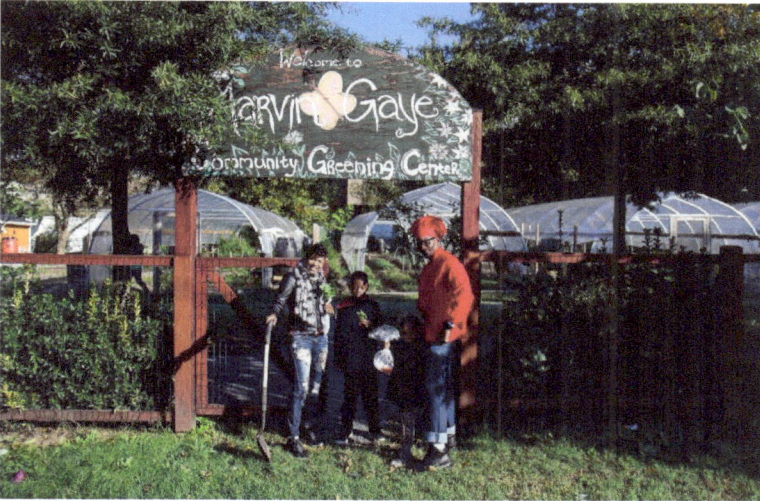

Antonio Ford

This book is dedicated to your family

from The Food Lord family

Hi kids…

Did you know before foods make it to the grocery store they have to grow on a farm first?

Well, let's hit the farm and grow some food. Let's plant a garden with The Food Lord and Family.

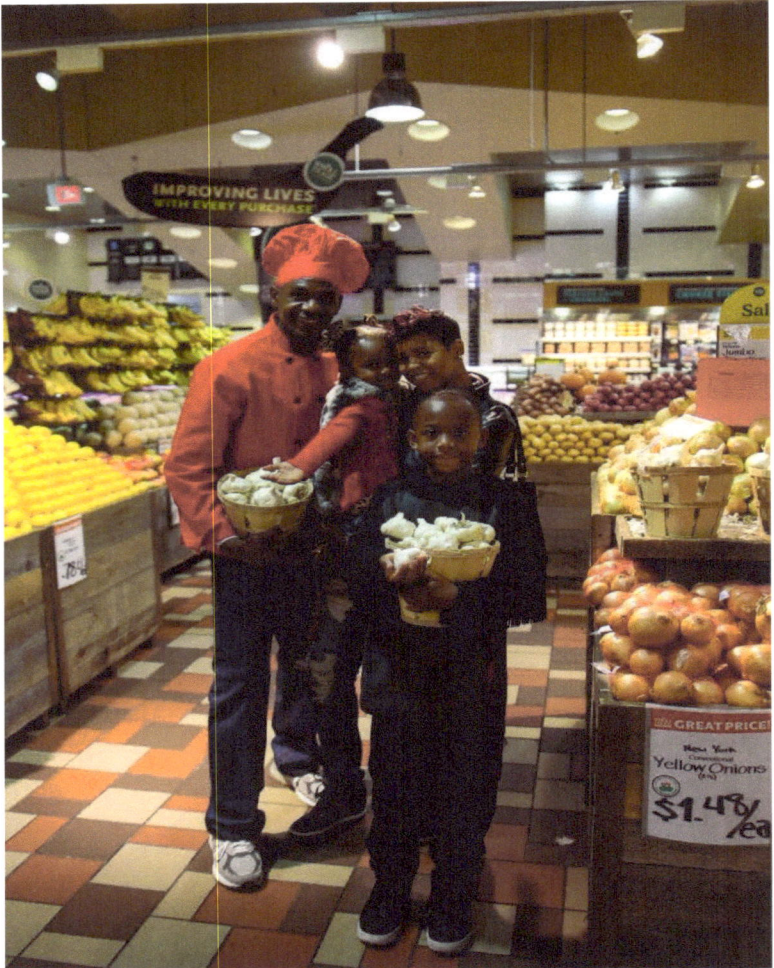

We are Team Ford and I am "The Food Lord." That is my wife, "Mother Food Lord," my son, Seven, and my daughter, Serenity.

Today, we will be planting Swiss Chard and Watermelon seeds.

Growing food takes patience, time, plenty of water and sun. If we can practice patience, in time those once planted seeds will grow. First, let's plant some Watermelon seeds, Serenity.

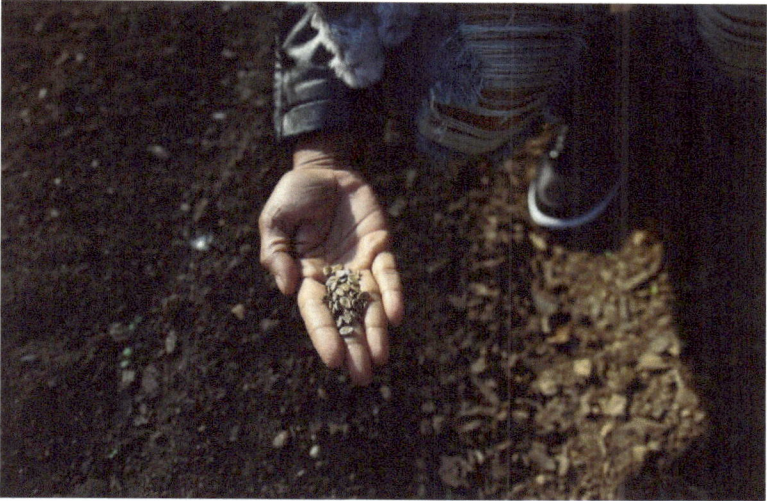

Serenity – I love yummy, delicious, juicy watermelons. They are rich in antioxidants. You may not know, but vitamin C is antioxidant. Don't forget this, okay?

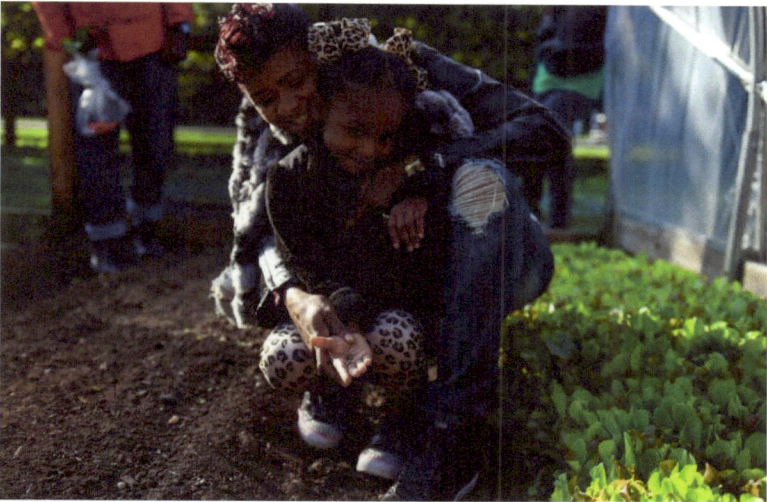

Where is Seven? Here I am over in the Swiss Chard section. This is Swiss Chard. It is very beautiful and ready to be picked. Swiss Chard is rich with protein and antioxidants which is excellent for growing children like me and my sister.

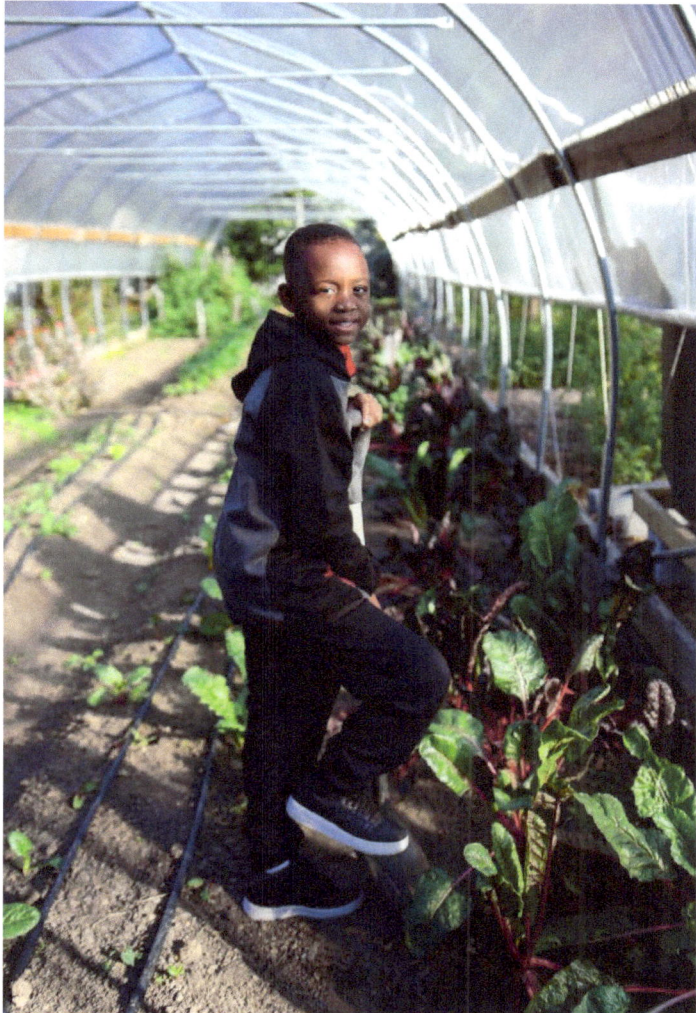

Serenity – You know what I love about Swiss Chard? It tastes great! I love to eat it raw, in a salad, or steamed! This superfood is so beautiful in color. One little secret about growing Swiss Chard, never pick the center stalk as the leaves continue to reproduce very quickly.

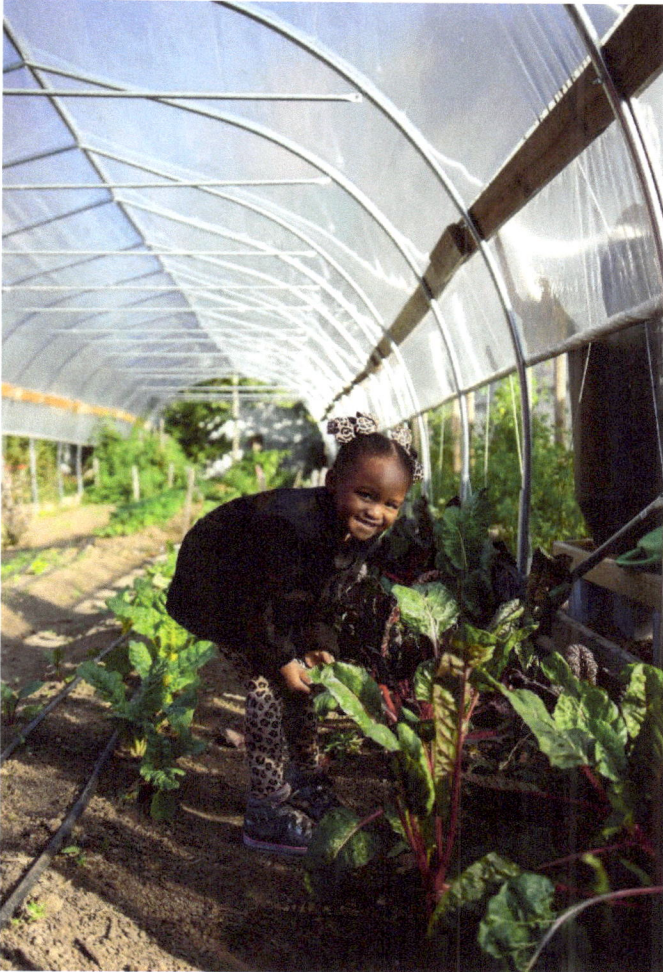

My name is Melanin. I watch over the garden to keep unwanted animals from eating up everything! I love my job watching over the garden. I also love to spend time with Seven. He plays with me and rubs me too!

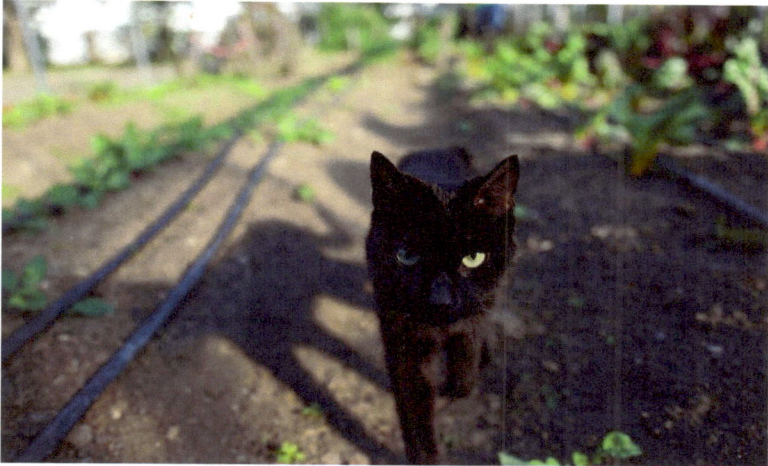

A Superfood like Swiss Chard is hard to find in grocery stores because it doesn't ship well. Growing it yourself allows it to tolerate hot as well as cool temperatures. If it freezes, it will die.

Children, ask your parents to grow food and watch how much fun it brings.

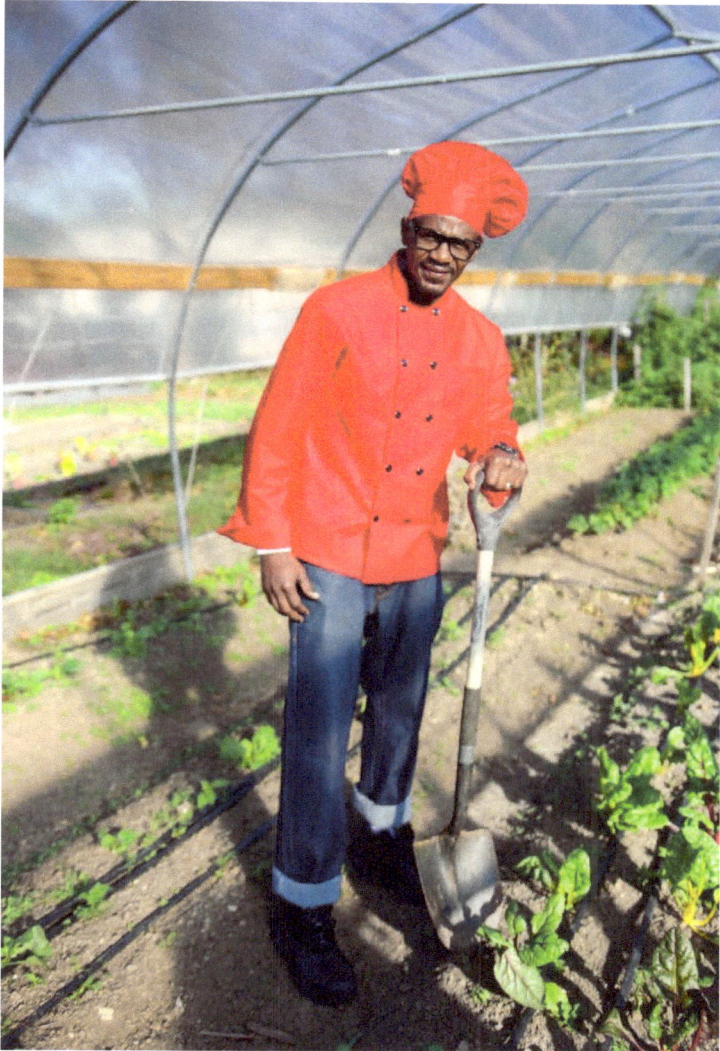

Remember these few words ... Eating from a healthy garden brings tremendous benefit. Eat for health, love yourself, plant a garden then exchange foods with other gardeners. Foods are a great way to make friends and keep them! It all starts here inside the Earth and it grows like this Swiss Chard.

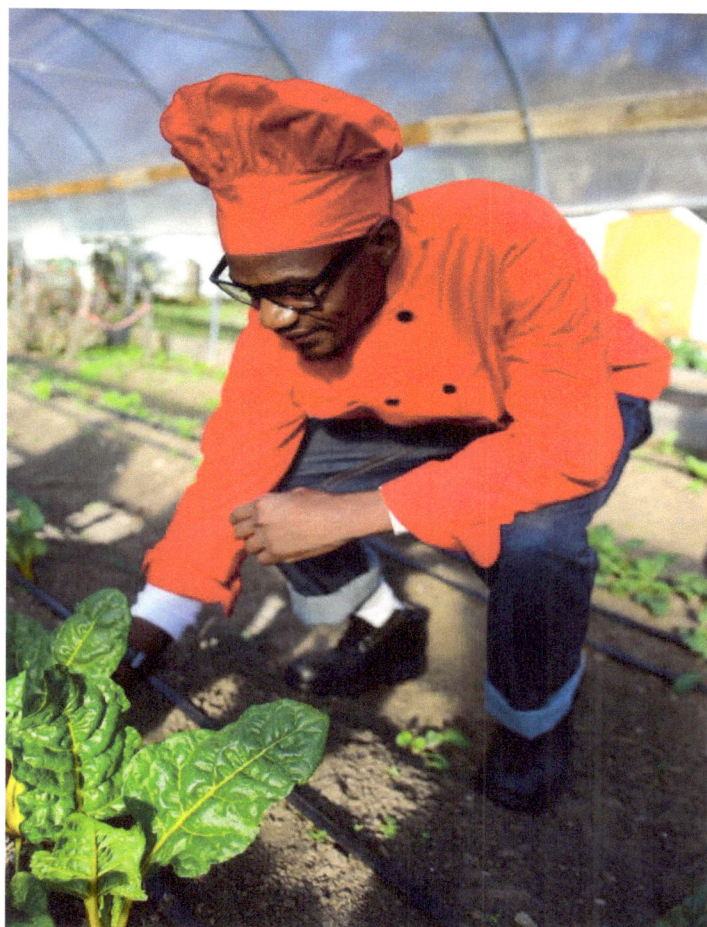

The End

www.ingramcontent.com/pod-product-compliance
Lightning Source LLC
Chambersburg PA
CBHW041442290326

41933CB00034B/47